BECOMING A
Woman
of
Purpose

— Lessons from —
Godly Women

Vicki L. Darbonne, MBA

Beyond The Book Media, LLC
Alpharetta. GA
www.beyondthebookmedia.com

ISBN: 978-1-966430-26-1 (Print)

TABLE OF CONTENTS

DEDICATION

---

*I dedicate this book to my mom, Vivian Escott.
Thank you for sacrificing, inspiring, and encouraging
me to pursue my dreams.*

*In Loving Memory of my grandmothers,
Mattie P Sherrod planted a seed of faith in me to follow
Christ.*

Mattie Fore encouraged me to read the Book of Psalms.

---

*"Apply your heart to instruction and your
ears to words of knowledge."*

-Proverbs 23:12

INTRODUCTION

"As the Father has loved me, so I have loved you. Abide in my love."
John 15:9

You are a crown of beauty and a royal diadem in the hand of the Lord (Isaiah 62:3). You are so loved, and God created you with special qualities and characteristics, and He has a specific purpose for us to fulfill.

I'm glad you decided to pick this book. My goal is that you glean from the exercises and lessons and examine your life to see if you are walking in your purpose. Remember, we were created in God's image to be loved by Him and to have fellowship with Him. Jesus' death fulfilled God's promise to deal with the curse of sin and death.

"Jesus Christ, who gave himself for our sins to rescue us from
this present evil age..."
Galatians 1:4

As women, we need to know our purpose in God because it provides a foundational sense of identity, value, and direction in life, allowing us to live with fulfillment by aligning our actions with God's design for us. That is, our gifts, talents, and abilities to serve others, show compassion, and reflect God's love in the world.

As a little girl, one of the many lessons I learned from my grandmother was to listen to what she told me. She planted the seed of my wanting to know about Christ. My grandmother could not read, yet she had the knowledge and wisdom to instill in me the importance of having God in my life. I learned to always seek the Lord in everything I do.

As for you, reader, do you know your purpose in life? In the Bible, *it says, For I know the plans I have for you, "declares the Lord, plans to prosper you and not harm you, plans to give you hope and a future"* (Jeremiah 29:11).

CHAPTER 1

Love Never Fails

*"Love never fails. But whether there are prophecies, they will fail;
whether there are tongues, they will cease; whether there is knowledge,
it will vanish away. For we know in part, and we prophesy in part. But
when that which is perfect has come, then that which is in
part will be done away."*
1 Corinthians 13:8-10

What is love in action? The Bible reveals how Jesus demonstrated compassion and care through His words and deeds. He calls us to love one another and provides clear examples of how to put that love into action. Ultimately, Jesus' sacrificial love for the world is the greatest example of love in action.

*"For God so loved the world, that he gave His only begotten Son, that
whosoever believeth in Him should not perish,
but have everlasting life."*
John 3:16

Christ died for the ungodly, and those who are united with Him through faith are justified in Him. As Paul explains, "He made Him who knew no sin to be sin for us, that we might become the righteousness of God in Him." From this perspective, Christ's work restores humanity to a right relationship with God. Scripture also teaches us to offer hope and encouragement through words, actions, and support in times of need.

My dear sister-in-Christ, Vernita, 70 years young, is a Godly woman I love like a big sister. Recently, she was diagnosed with Alzheimer's disease, a condition that disproportionately affects African Americans. According to the CDC, African Americans are twice as likely as older white adults to develop Alzheimer's or another form of dementia and are less likely to receive a timely diagnosis. This disease brings profound changes—in memory, thinking, and behavior—yet through it all, Vernita's spirit and faith continue to shine, inspiring everyone around her."

Despite her diagnosis, Vernita's Godly character continues to leave a lasting impact on everyone around her—her family, her sisters-in-Christ, and her husband, Bernard Aikens, a retired Army Colonel. Bernard cherishes the many memorable moments they've shared since they first met, moments filled with love, faith, and unwavering companionship. *The man said,*

> *"This is now bone of my bones*
> *and flesh of my flesh;*
> *she shall be called 'woman,'*
> *for she was taken out of man."*

> *That is why a man leaves his father and mother and is united to his wife, and they become one flesh.*
> *Genesis 2:23-24*

When Two Shall Become One

"And the two shall become one flesh; so, then they are no longer two, but one flesh. Therefore, what God has joined together, let no man separate."
Mark 10:8-9

One will find it if one looks for the good; if one looks for a Godly wife, one will find her. After my wife of 23 years passed away from colon cancer, I was undoubtedly lost because the center of my universe was taken away after a year-long battle with the dreaded "C" word that scares all of us, even those with strong faith. God is a good God who takes care of His own in ways we can't even comprehend, such as when two Alpha personalities come together—one from military service and the other from the corporate ladder of success. In June 2000, I moved to my last active-duty assignment as the Professor of Military Science at Jackson State University, an established Historically Black College and University (HBCU) in Jackson, MS.

After almost ten years outside the U.S. and away from my culture, my time at JSU was outstanding. While thriving on the secular side of my life, I sought membership at the South Madison Church of Christ in Ridgeland, MS. There, I taught adult classes, served the Lord's Supper, ushered, and immersed myself in Christian service.

As I began my new journey as a widow, I made a commitment to God and myself that if He blessed me with a Godly woman, I would marry again. At South Madison, I met a Christian lady named Caroline Montgomery and her husband, Bert Montgomery. Caroline and Bert, both Vietnam veterans, often shared their military experiences with me. After seeing me actively involved in the church for about a year, Caroline believed I might be the right Christian man for her unmarried sister, Vernita Ann Lauderdale.

In September 2000, Vernita visited Caroline and Bert and attended Wednesday night Bible class. She wore a beautiful pink outfit that showcased her many wonderful qualities as an athletic-looking woman. I was seated about three rows in front of her when I turned around and saw my future wife. After she returned to Dallas, I asked Caroline who she was and if she would introduce us. Caroline, ever the caring sister, gave me Vernita's phone number and email address. I wrote a letter of introduction and asked to meet her the next time she visited Jackson and South Madison Church of Christ. Vernita responded to my email, and we quickly agreed to share our hopes and dreams during lengthy phone conversations. Our conversations flowed easily, revealing more similarities than differences.

By January 2001, we were traveling back and forth to attend church services at either Greenville Avenue Church of Christ (GACC) or South Madison Churches of Christ. Any opportunity to be together was acceptable, regardless of distance or weather. Since Shreveport, Louisiana, was approximately halfway between Dallas and Jackson, we often met there for church services. By May, we knew we were soulmates, and during a dinner at Steak & Ale in Jackson, I asked her to be my wife and presented her with an engagement ring. As our long-distance courtship continued, we decided to wed on May 26, 2002, after completing marriage counseling under the mentorship of Brother David Phillips, an elder at Greenville Avenue Church of Christ. We also asked Senior Minister Brother Shelton Gibbs III to preside over our wedding in the auditorium at GACC. While planning the wedding, I met many of Vernita's close Christian friends who loved her dearly. Among them were Brother Anthony and Pam Travis, Ernie and Vonda Douglass, and David and Deloris Myers. She also positively impacted the lives of her sisters-in-Christ: Vicki Darbonne, Sabrina Smith, Barbara Culpepper, and Janet Threadgill. There are many others whose names I cannot remember; God knows your love for Vernita.

On May 26, 2002, God blessed us with a beautiful day. My son, Bradford L.K. Aikens, and stepson, Vince P. Lingner, flew into Dallas the day before and settled into their hotel. Vernita's brothers, Bruce, Michael, and David Lauderdale, arrived for the wedding along with her sisters Caroline, Denise, Judie, and Lisa, who were all preparing for the ceremony. Bruce Lauderdale served as the best man, and Bradford Aikens was the groomsman. Everything was set as I handed Bradford the rings the day before. At 2:00 PM on May 26, 2002, guests at GACC eagerly awaited my bride's entrance. When the wedding song began and the doors opened, the most beautiful woman walked toward me, escorted by her brother, Bruce Lauderdale. Brother Shelton Gibbs III eloquently emphasized that marriage is a covenant with God that we both took to love and care for each other in sickness and health. As part of the proceedings, I read an original poem about marriage that I had written specifically for Vernita, capturing my lifelong commitment to her and to God.

After the wedding, we enjoyed a week-long cruise through the Western Caribbean Islands and Puerto Rico. Since we had not lived together with my work in Jackson and Vernita's job in Dallas, we decided upon my retirement to take off for a year and work through actually living together. With a foundation in faith, we overcame all early marriage adversaries.

As a couple, we enjoyed serving the Lord, working in several ministries, including the nursing home ministry, along with our brothers and sisters-in-Christ. We'd sing, share the gospel, have communion, give encouragement, and pray with the residents. Afterwards, we all engaged in discussions at Anthony and Pam's home with Ernie and Vonda, and Greg and Vicki.

Currently, we have been married for 23 years, and she is a cherished part of my life. Due to the ravages of Alzheimer's disease, she now lives in a senior living community. Still, her Christian brothers and sisters and I show our love for her through daily and weekly visits. I appreciate the family of saints at Greenville Avenue Church of Christ.

When He saw the crowds, he went upon the mountain, and after He sat down, His disciples came to Him. Then, He began to teach them, saying:

"Blessed are the poor in spirit, for the kingdom of heaven is theirs.
Blessed are those who mourn,
for they will be comforted.
Blessed are the humble,
for they will inherit the earth.
Blessed are those who hunger and thirst for righteousness,
for they will be filled.
Blessed are the merciful,
for they will be shown mercy,
Blessed are the pure in heart,
for they will see God.
Blessed are the peacemakers,
for they will be called sons of God.

Blessed are those who are persecuted because of righteousness,
for the kingdom of heaven is theirs.
Matthew 5:1-10

Twenty-three years ago, I met Vernita, a smart, educated, sophisticatedly dressed, career-focused woman with a strong sense of self and ambition, at church through Beverly and Rebecca. Vernita and I always called them Mary and Martha, two sweet, wonderful sisters in Christ. Vernita shared with me about joining her book club, and I met a plethora of wonderful sisters in Christ enjoying a common bond in reading. Our sweet sister Karen B. so graciously accepted the baton to carry on the book club, and member growth is on the rise.

In this season of Alzheimer's, Vernita has many sisters in Christ who love her dearly. Vernita had an impact on all of us, and each of us is sharing our precious moments with her.

Surprisingly, Vernita and I were both planning our weddings in 2002. Vonda organized her bridal shower, while Karen R. beautifully prepared mine—it was a wonderful celebration. Vonda even created a lovely photo album of the event. This was an exciting and joyful time for both of us. I married Greg in April at the church, wearing my beautiful wedding gown. When Vernita married Bernard, she also wore a stunning wedding dress.

We got to know Bernard and Vernita even better when Greg and I began visiting nursing homes weekly with Anthony and Pam, Ernie and Vonda, and Paige and Destiny. After visiting Anthony and Pam's home, we often enjoyed the delicious pork steaks Anthony grilled. We shared many wonderful moments serving in ministry together.

Interestingly, Vernita was the reason Ernie and Vonda became a couple—it's truly a sweet love story. Vernita and I also share a common bond: our love for reading. She once invited me to join her book club, Reading Between the Lines, which meets at the end of each month. I gladly accepted. Indeed, Vernita truly loves to read.

Since Vernita worked at Alcatel-Lucent, we both worked in Plano and often met for lunch to catch up, which I always enjoyed. I love her dearly. One memorable trip I'll never forget was traveling with Vernita and her sisters, Lisa and Judy, to San Antonio for Judy's son's graduation at Lackland Air Force Base — it was such a special and unforgettable experience we shared together.

Vernita has always had such a caring heart. When Greg fractured his hip and was recovering at home, she stepped right in to help. I would prepare his meals in the crockpot before heading to work, and Vernita made sure he was taken care of throughout the day — checking on him and bringing his meals while he was confined to bed. Her kindness and dependability made that difficult time so much easier for us.

Sister Wright is truly gifted in so many ways. I still remember when Vernita showed me a beautiful, large, knitted blanket of love she had made for them — every stitch seemed to carry her warmth and care. During Greg's recovery, she also brought over her mouth-watering, "fall-off-the-bone" barbecue ribs — tender, flavorful, and so delicious they practically melted in your mouth. Her thoughtfulness and talent brought both comfort and joy during that time."

Vernita and I often went shopping together, sharing laughter and meaningful conversations. She had a special love for her plants, and I always admired her classy, sophisticated sense of style. Her home reflected that same grace — beautifully decorated, warm, and inviting. Around that time, Greg and I became Care Group leaders, with Stephen and Gloria graciously passing the baton and sharing their wisdom and ministry experience. We began hosting Bible studies in our home, preparing meals and welcoming others into fellowship. Bernard and Vernita were always there, offering unwavering support. Spending more time serving alongside them in the nursing home ministry deepened our bond even further. As couples, we created many cherished memories — watching fireworks at Firewheel, attending the Gospel Campaign in downtown Dallas, and enjoying Bible study evenings where, more often than not, it was just the four of them — Stephen and Gloria, and Bernard and Vernita — faithfully by our side."

One day, Bernard and Greg led a Bible study with my Air Force buddy Mark, a retired SMSgt who later married his lovely wife, Tonia while Vernita and I listened and joined in the fellowship. I'll never forget the day Greg fractured his hip. Bernard and Vernita came to the hospital, and together we prayed, leaning on faith and each other for strength. Vernita has always held a special place in my heart. She listens with genuine care, offers wisdom without hesitation, and encourages you when the weight of life feels too heavy. Even now, her gentle words to 'keep on living' echo in my mind, reminding me to move forward with hope and grace.

Sometimes after Bible class, I'd slip into the car with Vernita and her sister, Lisa, and we'd make our way to McDonald's for coffee or tea. We'd sit there in the parking lot, cups warming our hands, sharing stories, laughter, and the little moments that quietly stitched our lives together. Those mornings became some of my sweetest memories."

Even when Vernita stepped away from the book club, Karen graciously carried the tradition forward, joined by Barbara, Janet, Patricia, and Marin—keeping the warmth, fellowship, and familiar rhythm of our gatherings alive. Over the years, our little circle blossomed into a lively group of ten to seventeen women, meeting on Saturdays at the end of each month. We were especially delighted when Anissa returned, her presence bringing a sense of homecoming to our discussions. To stay organized, we selected all our books for the year in advance, giving everyone time to prepare. Our meetings rotated from home to home—sometimes even spilling into cozy corners of local restaurants—where we shared more than the stories on the page. We shared laughter, honest conversations, and the kind of friendship that nourishes the soul.

One memorable highlight of our book club was when Patricia, a longtime member, hosted our very first Holiday Party in her beautiful home. We gathered together, and a group photo captured the joy of the moment — the ladies posed in front of a sparkling white Christmas tree, adorned with glittering ornaments, each of us holding our gifts and soaking in the warmth and happiness of being together."

Our book club has grown into so much more than a gathering to discuss books—it has become a sanctuary of friendship, trust, and love. I feel deeply grateful that Vernita invited me to join; her invitation has been a true blessing, not just for me, but for all the ladies who share in this journey. Watching the group grow over time, welcoming new members and the energy they bring, has been a joy. I treasure the countless moments of laughter, conversation, and support we've shared. Even now, in the face of Vernita's new diagnosis, we continue to gather, holding close the bond we've nurtured and the meaningful time we spend together." Each meeting is a reminder of the enduring joy, faith, and friendship that have carried us through life's seasons, and we cherish every precious moment we're blessed to spend together."

I cherished every walk with Vernita; when I arrived, she would jokingly ask, "Now, where you been?" and I'd reply, "Looking for you," and we'd laugh before heading out together. I also loved taking her on outings, like our trip to the Naval Air Station Joint Reserve Base in Fort Worth, with Beverly joining us. Visits with Vonda were always a delight—her delicious down-home southern meals, shopping excursions, and the style of braiding Vernita's hair left lasting memories. Vernita adored strolling through the rose gardens in Fort Worth and admiring the vibrant, elegant blooms at the Dallas Arboretum. I treasured capturing photos of her enjoying these moments, especially one of her gently rocking in Yvonne's chair, the breeze blowing softly, as we shared a quiet, peaceful time together. Another memory I hold close is a group photo Lisa's husband took of Vernita, Lisa, her brother, and me—a snapshot of joy and togetherness that felt truly beautiful.

Above all, God's presence shines beautifully through Vernita's life. Whether sitting or walking, she shares a deep and personal relationship with Him—she walks with Him, talks with Him, and knows she belongs to Him.

My time with Vernita has taught me to find joy in life's simple moments and to appreciate the small expressions of love that are often overlooked. When I hug her and kiss her cheek, her face lights up with joy. Although she may not always remember names or details, she never forgets how you make her feel. These precious moments with Vernita are memories I will always treasure in my heart.

"Love suffers long and is kind; love does not envy; love does not parade itself, is not puffed up; does not behave rudely, does not seek its own, is not provoked, thinks no evil, does not rejoice in iniquity, but rejoices in the truth; bears all things, believes all things, hopes all things, endures all things. Love never fails, but whether there are prophecies, they will fail; whether there are tongues, they will cease; whether there is knowledge, it will vanish away."
1 Corinthians 13:4-8

"And now abide faith, hope, love, these three; but the greatest of these is love."
1 Corinthians 13:13

Even in her season of Alzheimer's, Vernita's spirit shone brightly, a testament to her unwavering faith and clear understanding of her purpose in God. Beloved by her many sisters in Christ, she shared her gifts of communication, enthusiasm, support, and attentive listening—gifts that drew us together and strengthened our bond. As we gather to share our stories, our hearts overflow with gratitude for the love, joy, and inspiration she has poured into our lives—a legacy of grace and light that will remain with us forever.

Sister Rebecca T. shares a meeting with Vernita.

In my relationship with Vernita, I thank God for all our years of friendship and for having her as a dear sister in Christ. I will always cherish our fun and laughter while acting and clowning around. I pray that God continues to strengthen and bless her life. I love you dearly, my sister.

Sister Beverly D. shares her story of meeting Vernita.

I met Sis. Vernita in 1987 or 1988 at Hamilton Park Church of Christ, also known as Greenville Avenue Church of Christ. She was friendly and welcoming, and we participated in several singles activities together. Vernita, a career woman, worked for Electronic Data Systems

(EDS), an American multinational information technology and services company based in Plano, Texas. She was always professional while working at EDS, and through a program that selected a group of young people to go to London, England. She chose Damar and Wendy to participate in the program. They enjoyed traveling to another country, and this experience is one they will always cherish.

Sis. Vernita is very humble and eager to help her family and others. I'm so grateful to have her as my sister in Christ and a wonderful friend.

Sister Anissa A. expresses her heartfelt gratitude to Vernita.

I want to share my sincere appreciation for Vernita, whose kindness and wisdom have profoundly impacted my life. Years ago, when I first got married, Vernita took the time to offer me advice that has stayed with me ever since. She encouraged me to truly invest in my marriage and prioritize it, helping to lay the foundation for the strong and enduring relationship I am fortunate to have today. Vernita's warmth and generous spirit have touched so many people, and I am deeply thankful to know such a wonderful sister.

Sister Marinett B., who has passed on to glory, shared her story about Vernita.

I met Vernita when I joined the Book Club about 14 years ago. At first, I thought Vernita didn't like me because she had very little to say and didn't seem very friendly. It wasn't until I had my back operation in 2013 and she and Vicki Darbonne came to visit me that I realized she did care for me. Their visit was long and very comforting. Over the years, Vernita and I grew closer to the point that we decided to form our own little two-person visitation team. We chose to visit members who were homebound, as well as those in the hospital and rehab facilities. We picked members mentioned in our Church Bulletin. We went visiting after the Young at Heart Bible Study Class on Thursdays. Either she would drive, or I would, leaving our cars in the Church parking lot.

Vernita and I formed a two-person visitation team for about two years, which I named the Merry Visitors (M for Marinett and V for Vernita). We did this independently, without anyone directing or facilitating us. I found great joy in working with Vernita; she was easy to collaborate with, and we both had so much fun and fulfillment in this work. Vernita will always hold a positive place in my life for her foresight in establishing the Reading Between the Lines Book Club, where I not only met her but also other ladies who shared a passion for reading.

Sister Pam T. shares her thoughts about my dear friend, Vernita.

Vernita and I have been friends for over 30 years, and throughout that time, she has proven herself to be an exceptional individual and a cherished part of my life. We have enjoyed working together in various ministries over the years. I can confidently say that Vernita's dedication and ability to bring people together have always been remarkable. She knows how to strike the perfect balance between being fun and funny while staying serious and focused when needed to get the job done. Her work ethic and commitment are truly inspiring. In addition to our ministry work, Vernita and I worked together at EDS. Vernita worked in Payroll, and I worked in the Claims Department. During that time, we spent countless lunch breaks working out together and then returning to work. Those moments reflected Vernita's commitment to self-improvement and her ability to make everyday routines more enjoyable and memorable. Outside of work and ministry, I truly enjoyed spending time with Vernita. Whether hanging out, sharing stories, or simply enjoying each other's company, our time together was always meaningful and joyful. Vernita will always hold a special place in my life, and I am grateful for our bond. She is, and always will be, my friend.

Sister Delores L. Myers shares how she met Vernita.

I first met Vernita long ago after placing membership with Hamilton Park Church of Christ in the late '80s. I think one of our first outings together was a musical theater event. Vernita was a woman of character and very self-sufficient. She was educated, smart, witty, and funny, and loved laughing. A go-getter and hard worker, she owned real estate, got into investing, and was a dedicated employee. As a faithful church member, she loved to read, valued her health, and practiced healthy living. We also participated in many activities together with the singles' ministry.

Vernita and I would always have conversations centered around hair and exercise because we both understood the importance of exercise. Still, we also understood that we had to sacrifice something (perfect hair, at least that's how we saw it then) to improve and maintain our health. Vernita and I also started a workout class at the church building, and we would lead exercise classes for our sisters of the congregation. I don't remember how long we did that, but we both enjoyed it. Vernita and Bro. Phillips (one of our elders) taught the gospel to my husband, and he obeyed. They soon reintroduced us, and the rest is history. So, Vernita and Bro. Phillips is part of the reason David and I got together. Vernita and Bro. Phillips remained close and shared a special bond until he died in 2023.

I was also part of the original book club initiated by Vernita (I don't remember if she was the sole brain behind it). We named it "Reading Between the Lines," and I enjoyed the fellowship it offered. I used to be part of a group, but eventually stopped attending (I attributed that to having kids). However, if you are an avid reader, nothing stops you from reading continuously. Now that my kids are grown and gone, I have no excuses left. I always admired Vernita for NOT settling for just any guy. I believe she had decided (before meeting Bernard) that she might be single for the rest of her life—I think she was okay with that. But God had other plans.

I remember when Vernita and Bernard started dating; it was so lovely to see her with such a wonderful guy, and we were all happy for her. I was honored to be part of their special day (I was a hostess and pregnant with my second child). Look how God blessed her and Bernard with each other at that time. One day during COVID, after our congregation returned to the building, I was working at the entrance, helping to take temperatures, when I noticed Vernita and Bernard. There was something about her I couldn't quite put my finger on when our eyes met. I saw that blank stare, that look in her eyes I was all too familiar with—because my husband's mother had dementia, I sensed something was wrong. I didn't say anything to anyone about what I saw that day. Sometime after that,

I talked to Vernita and asked her about life, work, etc. Something seemed off about her responses to my questions regarding her work. She then told me about her diagnosis. I was heartbroken and couldn't believe what she was telling me. As the days went on, I noticed the changes.

I remember those times earlier when Vernita would talk about her mother living with this dreadful disease. She would talk about events and things, sometimes funny, serious, and sad. But of course, none of us would have guessed that Vernita would end up with dementia. Also, I gave Bernard a break and took Vernita with me for the day. We went to my daughter's high school track meet. It was a cold day in February, and we would return to the car to warm up. After we left the track meet, we went to eat. Now, her husband had put money in her purse to pay for her meal. When it was time to pay, she did not want me to say anything about going into her purse to pay for her meal. I'm sure she thought I was going to take her money. She also became agitated (which was probably too much; we were out for a long time). I paid for the meal to keep the peace, which was fine. My only regret is not getting her enough to help Bernard before she started declining. I will cherish our friendship. I vividly remember the laughs we would share—she enjoyed laughing. And I think she loved popcorn as much as I do. Thank you, Vernita, for sharing your life with me.

Sister Sheryl D. shares when she first met Vernita in the 1980s.

Shortly after I moved here in 1984, we connected at Hamilton Park Church of Christ through various activities and work areas, as we were both active members. She was single when I first met her. Vernita was always friendly, warm, and outgoing. She made me feel welcome from the start. I enjoyed our conversations immensely. She was very spiritual and incredibly intelligent. I never walked away from a conversation with her without learning something new. Vernita had a natural talent for bringing people together. She helped me get to know more people, which meant a lot to me, especially since I initially knew only a few people in the congregation.

A few years later, I got to know her even better when she started hosting black hair sessions at home. Vernita, who was married now, invited sisters to come together and taught us about different hair products for our specific hair types, how to properly care for our hair, black hairstyles, and more. We learned a lot, had fun, and enjoyed great fellowship along the way. These sessions allowed all of us to get to know each other better. Although I don't see her as often now, I always greet her with a warm smile whenever I do.

Sister Phyllis T. shares her story of when she first met Vernita Aiken, also known as Vernita Lauderdale, in the fall of 1989.

I worked at Presbyterian Hospital of Dallas alongside Ava Booker, who was Ava Davis then. Ava knew I had been seeking God for a while and shared some of the things she had learned as a member of the Church of Christ. She told me she could arrange a Bible study with some church members. That's when I first met Vernita. Every week, Vernita would come to my apartment to study the Bible with me, accompanied by Elder David Phillips and Deloris Meyers. While I don't remember all the details from 35 years ago, I do remember Vernita's beautiful smile and her consistent presence. Because of my interactions with all three of them, I was baptized in late October 1989 at Hamilton Park Church of Christ.

After my baptism, Vernita's unique and inviting voice stayed with me, encouraging me to participate in church events and helping me feel a part of the body. I am deeply grateful to all three, especially to Vernita, for her vital role in teaching me the gospel.

Big Sis! Our big sister Vernita has been a tremendous inspiration to us over the years. Ernie met her in the mid-80s and formed an instant bond. She became his big sister, encouraging and guiding him through some tough times as a young single man. When I met Ernie in the late 80s, he introduced Vernita to me as his big sister. She quickly sized me up and gave him the stamp of approval. Her advice and opinions were always important because he knew she would tell him the godly truth about everything. Vernita was raised in a Christian household, drawing her strength, knowledge, and faith in God and from her father, who she often quoted as saying, "He didn't play." She encouraged us throughout our courtship and naturally became my big sister. When Ernie and I faced little bumps in our relationship, Vernita was always there to shake us off, push us back into the ring, and remind us, "Hang in there; it's going to be okay."

We love Vernita so much. She has always been classy, smart, funny, beautiful, and independent—full of strength, knowledge, love, compassion, courage, and unwavering faith.

Vernita's illness has caused her to hit a bump in the road, but just as she never gave up on us, we continue to pray for a healing miracle. She is still so full of life, and that is a true blessing, especially considering how long she has been battling her illness. God is good. Thank you, Big Sis. We will forever be grateful to you and will always be here for you.

Sister Karen E. shares her first meeting with Vernita in the summer of 91.

Her aunt, Sojourner, and my mother were best friends when we lived in Germany in the 70s. When I moved to Dallas in 91, my mother kept in touch with Ms. Sojourner; she told my mother that she had some nieces that lived in Dallas and she was going to visit them; my mother had me meet Ms. Sojourner at her niece's apartment which turned out to be Vernita, we quickly got a long, and Vernita began a VBS with me, and Delores Meyers was the silent partner. After about three weeks of Bible study, I was baptized on a Tuesday evening as I was ready to accept Christ as the living Son of God. It was about 9 p.m. on a Tuesday when Vernita contacted Bro. David Phillips to baptize me.

Sister Karen B. shares her story about Vernita.

I first met Vernita in 2007 at a book club meeting, thanks to my dear friend and angel, Cheryl Rainey, who invited me to join. Cheryl had mentioned this wonderful group of Christian women who gathered once a month to read and discuss books. I was intrigued, yet unsure if I could actually finish an entire book each month. When I attended my first meeting, it was like magic. The women were so warm and welcoming. I shared my concerns about not being able to finish a book in time, but they reassured me. They said it was okay if I couldn't read it all—just come for the fellowship and read as much as possible. When I met Vernita, I knew right away that she was special. She was incredibly passionate about the book club and what it represented. Vernita was the leader and founder of the group, and I had never seen anyone so organized and well-equipped to oversee a group. She commanded the room with such ease and grace.

Vernita brought a bag of books, a notebook with extra readings, a list of previous books, and an outline for the entire year's reading schedule. I was so impressed that the book club even had a name—Reading Between the Lines—and a logo. Later, we were each given a book bag featuring the logo, and every month had a different theme or category, including Trailblazers, Black Authors, Mystery, Romance, Spiritual, Classic, and Autobiographies. Vernita consistently arrived at each meeting well-prepared and on time. She had discussion questions ready and set the tone for the meeting.

I will always be grateful for this group. Surprisingly, I managed to read the entire book each month. In fact, I looked forward to not only socializing (and we did a lot of that) but also discussing the book. In honor of Vernita, we have continued the book club and her vision. These women are now and will always be my sisters and friends. Thanks to the incredible woman who started this group, we are all now lovers of books and avid readers. Thank you, Vernita, for your friendship and for bringing us together. May God bless you and keep you.

Sister Janet T. shares about our friend Vernita.

Proverbs 27:17 (KJV) states, "Iron sharpeneth iron; so a man sharpeneth the countenance of his friend." This Bible verse reminds me of my wonderful friend Vernita. She was straightforward and provided the best advice when it was needed. Vernita also had a warm and engaging personality, and we loved chatting about various topics, especially recipes. I met her in 2000 when I joined Greenville Avenue Church of Christ. She had a clever idea to start a book club and invited me to join, which I happily accepted. That was over 20 years ago, and we had such a great time picking out books and sharing our thoughts with the group. I fondly remember the time I was selecting hardwood flooring for my home. Vernita was among the few friends who truly understood my style and lifestyle. I showed her several samples, and we had a great conversation about the pros and cons of each option. With her help, I chose the perfect hardwood floor, which I still enjoy today!

Sister Patricia R. shares her story about Vernita.

I first met Vernita while working in the tape room. She came by to buy a tape of the sermon and introduced herself. She mentioned that she was one of the teachers or teacher's aides (I can't remember which) for the 6th-grade girls' Wednesday night Bible class. My daughter, Endia, was in that class. She told me she was impressed with my daughter because of her kindness. From then on, we chatted whenever we saw each other, especially when she visited the tape room. I truly got to know her when I joined the book club. I noticed that although she often appeared stern and no-nonsense, she had a wonderful sense of humor and was very kind. I appreciated her straightforwardness and leadership in the book club. I believe we connected well and had some similarities. I was heartbroken when she left the book club without knowing why she departed. Once I learned about her diagnosis, it saddened me to think that she would soon not remember who I was and that the friendship and sisterly affection we shared would be lost. I miss her dearly and pray that God blesses her as she navigates this stage of her life.

Sister Barbara C. shares her story back in probably '86 or '87, when Vernita met my stepmother, Sandra.

There was a group of 4 that Brother Patrick Worthey lovingly called the "Fly Girls": Vernita Lauderdale at the time, Angela Greene, Rita Jackson, and Sandra Culpepper. Vernita gave Sandra a Bible study along with Brother Phillips and a friend of ours who had introduced Sandra and Vernita. They went to all the single activities together and became lifelong friends. It was through that friendship that I came to know Vernita. I wasn't baptized and added to the church until July 5, 1991. But I had known Vernita shortly after she and Sandra met. One Sunday in the early 90s, Vernita and I talked, and we realized we shared a love of reading and liked some of the same authors. We exchanged some books and then came up with the idea of starting the book club. I came up with the name, which was voted on at one of the meetings. That's how we got our start.

Sister Sabrina S. shares her story of Vernita at the Greenville Avenue Church of Christ in 1999.

A mutual friend introduced us, and we connected right away. Vernita loved working with young people and served as a mentor to many young ladies at Greenville Ave and in her work community. One of her favorite sayings was, "How do you know it won't work if you haven't put much effort into trying?" Vernita and I had a lot in common, including a love for reading. She often said, "The demise of most folks is that they won't open a book." Because we shared a passion for reading, we created a book club to introduce others to our love of literature. The book club didn't have a name for a couple of years and eventually became known as "Reading Between the Lines." Although neither of us is active anymore, the book club continues under the leadership of Karen Bright. Vernita and I often took off on Saturdays to go dream house hunting. Our trips included finding model homes to explore and sharing our "expertise" on the details of the houses needed to attract potential buyers like us. Vernita's sense of humor and quick comebacks were top-notch. Whenever I faced a conflict with a co-worker, I would call her for advice, and she consistently provided me with the perfect professional words to share with my difficult colleague.

Sister Gloria R. recalls first meeting Vernita back in 2002 when she and Bernard had just gotten married.

My husband, Stephen, and I were the leaders of Care Group 1, and Bernard and Vernita became our Care Group assistants. I remember visiting their home for a delicious dinner, where we ate, talked, and got to know each other better. This marked the beginning of a beautiful relationship. We worked together to care for and meet the needs of families in our Care Group. We took turns hosting activities in our homes, such as Bible studies, attended bowling outings, and provided meals for members who had lost loved ones or were ill. Vernita is beautiful inside and out. Before being diagnosed with Alzheimer's, she was an avid reader and had a wonderful sense of humor. We shared a career path in real estate, both being Realtors. I will never forget the last time we talked for about three hours in my office; she shared stories about her childhood and upbringing, revealing so much about herself that I never knew during the 20+ years we had known each other.

CHAPTER 2

Pearls of Wisdom

"Her mouth speaks wisdom, and loving instruction is on her tongue."
Proverbs 31:26

Have you ever carried life lessons from your grandmother into adulthood? One early sunny morning, I heard my aunt Susan gently waking my grandmother, Mattie Pearl, for church. It was an early sunny morning when I heard my auntie walk into her bedroom. "Momma! Momma, you overslept for church." I woke up to the sound of my aunt gently waking my grandmother for church. Momma! Momma! My eyes were closed when I heard her walk down the hall. Listening to the sound of her slippers fade down the hall, I realized with a sinking feeling that my grandmother had passed.

Every weekend, I would take the subway to visit my grandmother and go to church with her. I treasured those moments in her company—her gentle words, her laughter, and the life lessons she shared about how to carry myself as a young lady. The night before, I had fallen asleep on her sofa bed by the window while she dozed peacefully in her own bed. That morning, sunlight streamed softly through the windows, warming the room and filling me with memories of our late-night conversations and the laughter we shared watching a John Wayne movie.

When my aunt called me, I slowly opened my eyes and saw her room bathed in golden light. Tears filled my eyes as they fell onto my cheeks, and I caught sight of her baby blue church hat hanging delicately on the corner of the dresser mirror—a small emblem of her grace and faith. As I prepared to leave, I lingered at her side, watching her rest peacefully, my aunt gently holding my hand. I was only twelve, yet my heart overflowed with love, memories, and disbelief of her passing.

Even now, I carry those mornings, those conversations, and that laughter in my heart. They remind me to cherish every moment and every person in life. I am profoundly grateful to God for allowing Mattie Pearl Sherrod to share her wisdom, her love, and her light with me, gifts I will carry forever.

It was the winter of 1972, and I was six years old when I stepped off the Greyhound bus into the snowy streets of New York, holding my mother's hand and walking alongside my brother, Marvin. One of the most enduring lessons I learned from her was the power of prayer. Every night, she would guide us on our knees, teaching us the Lord's Prayer, instilling in me a faith that has carried me through life.

I was born Vicki Lynn Escott in Birmingham, Alabama. We moved away with our parents, Walter and Vivian, leaving behind the familiar faces I'd known. Though I was too young to fully understand it then, that move marked the beginning of a new chapter.

My father had promised to come for us, and years later, he did. I still remember the day he arrived in Brooklyn, standing tall and smiling as he handed me a Bible and said softly, 'Make sure you read this.' It was more than a gift — it was a seed of faith he planted in my heart. Not long after, he arranged for us to visit him in Cleveland, Ohio, where Marvin and I would meet our baby sister for the first time. That moment marked not just a reunion but the beginning of understanding the quiet strength and love that defined him.

Marvin and I were overjoyed to be reunited with our grandmother, Mattie—affectionately known as 'Muah'—along with our aunts, uncles, and cousins. My father beamed with pride as he introduced me to my bright and spirited cousin, Gwendolyn Marie, whom I lovingly call today, 'sister cuz.' I can still see her now, laughing as she spun a bucket of water upside down, the water somehow staying inside—a little miracle to me. Those days were filled with wonder and warmth, moments of laughter and discovery that would linger in my heart long after childhood faded."

Little did I know that years later, in 1988, Gwen and her husband

Gus, both Marines, Marvin in the Army, and I in the Air Force, would fold the American flag 13 times in the precise triangular pattern at my father's funeral. "My father, Walter Escott Jr., a Vietnam veteran, carried the unseen weight of post-traumatic stress disorder, yet he remained a man of extraordinary gifts—brilliant with numbers, skilled with his hands, and moved by a quiet love for music. He could take a car apart and put it back together as effortlessly as he could teach us a game of chess and checkers, each moment becoming more than a lesson—it was his way of connecting, of showing love in the only language he knew. He left us a legacy of courage and love — one deeply intertwined with service, faith, and the desire to live with purpose.

Growing up in New York, my world shifted when I went to live with my grandmother, aunts, and cousins in a lively four-bedroom apartment in Harlem. The air was always buzzing with energy — children laughing in the streets, music spilling from open windows, and neighbors greeting one another from stoops. Yet beneath that rhythm of community was another pulse — one marked by the harsh realities of gang activity and the growing drug epidemic of the 1970s. Harlem was both beautiful and bruised, a place where resilience was learned early, and hope became a quiet act of courage.

As a Gen Xer and one of the latchkey kids, my childhood was woven into the streets of the city, where freedom meant staying out until the streetlights flickered on. Our days were spent hopping through hopscotch, calling out 'Simon Says,' and chasing each other in freeze tag, while I raced my bright orange Road Runner bike through the park, laughter bubbling until our cheeks ached. Those carefree afternoons—brimming with friendship, joy, and the simple pleasures of childhood—became the heartbeat of my youth, shaping a spirit of adventure and independence that lingered long after the sun went down."

One sweltering summer afternoon, I remember jumping Double Dutch with my friends, mesmerized by the sun glinting off Tina's brand-new white PRO-Keds. They seemed to shimmer with every step, and when I asked, she smiled shyly and said her boyfriend had bought them. But one day, Tina didn't come back. We waited, jump ropes in hand, our hearts full of hope, only to later learn that her boyfriend had lured her into a world no child should ever face. The emptiness she left behind settled deep in my heart, a piercing reminder that childhood innocence is fragile.

Despite the harsh realities of crime and heroin in my surroundings, summer days held joy—running through the spray of water from the opened fire hydrants and attending block parties with music blasting in the background, listening to Earth, Wind & Fire and Kool & the Gang's Summer Madness. What began in the Bronx with DJs spinning turntables grew into vibrant block parties that swept through Harlem and New York City, filling the streets with hip-hop, laughter, and a powerful sense of community—memories that still echo with joy today.

My fondest childhood memories were sitting on the stoop, chatting with my friend Patricia, one of the cool older sisters on the block. She and the others wore the fashion of the '70s—platform boogie shoes, bell-bottom pants, miniskirts, and styled afros or sleek ponytails. The stoop was more than just a set of stairs; it was our gathering place, where hot summer days were spent sharing stories, talking about school, and discussing the latest R&B groups.

One afternoon, everything changed. I came home from school to see our block on Eyewitness News Channel 7. My heart sank as I learned that Patricia had been found murdered in her car, and we later learned her boyfriend had tried to drag her into a dark life of prostitution. The grief cut even deeper because Morningside Park, just across the street from my window, had been our playground—lush green trees, steep hills, swings, and baseball fields where we played freeze tag, rolled down hills, and raced our bikes.

Every time I sat on the stoop afterward, I felt Patricia's absence keenly, missing the laughter, the chatter, and the simple joy of those carefree moments we had shared. Back then, our social network was built on real, in-person connections, where friendships were tangible and lasting. Today, many measure connection by the number of online friends they've never met, and the depth of true human interaction feels lost. The world may have changed, but the memory of those days—the friendships, the games, and the bonds we formed—remains etched in my heart,

When I was nine, I spent countless afternoons playing jacks with Jeanette while munching on sunflower seeds. We lived in the same seven-story apartment building at 272 Manhattan Avenue, and our days were filled with Double Dutch, freeze tag, hopscotch, and endless laughter. I prided myself on mastering the 'twosies' round of jacks. Whenever the ice cream truck music rang out, we would shout, 'THE ICE CREAM MAN IS COMING!' and sprint for our treats—my strawberry crunch bar in hand, Jeanette's red, white, and blue bomb pop smeared all over her face and arms.

But one day in class, when the teacher stepped out to get a box of chalks, I witnessed Jeanette and some classmates bullying a girl named Sabrina—kicking her chair, knocking down her books, and hurling cruel names. They urged me to kick Sabrina's bathroom stall door, and for a moment, I obeyed. Then, my grandmother's voice echoed in my mind: 'Do unto others as you would have them do unto you.' I felt a pang of shame and realized how wrong it was.

From that day forward, I chose a different path. I stopped hanging out with Jeanette and forged a friendship with Sabrina instead. Over the school year, I watched Jeanette get into fights and trouble, and I understood, even as a child, the importance of treating others with kindness and surrounding myself with people who shared the same values. This lesson profoundly shaped my character into adulthood. The Bible also reminds us to be mindful of the company we keep. *"Do not be misled: Bad company corrupts good character"* (1 Corinthians 15:1).

My grandmother, Mattie Pearl, was born in Birmingham, Alabama, and became a young widow raising seven children during the Jim Crow era, without the conveniences we take for granted today. She was a woman of remarkable strength and discipline, never one for gossip, and often reminded us, 'If you don't have anything nice to say, don't say anything.' Observant and protective, she always knew when something was wrong. She sacrificed endlessly and endured hardships, trusting that only God could carry her through those challenging times.

Grandma shaped me profoundly as a child. She was loving and caring, yet ruled with an iron hand. When she gave instructions, they were to be followed without question, or there would be consequences. I still remember her unyielding breakfast rule: no one went out to play until every last spoonful of oatmeal was eaten. Her discipline was tempered by love, and her guidance instilled in me a respect for perseverance, faith, and the strength of character that defined her life.

One important lesson she taught was to always listen. One day, I sneaked off with my cousins to the park despite her instructions to stay near the stoop. Grandma was sitting on the bench talking to a lady and saw us. She angrily said, "Didn't I tell you to stay by the stoop?" My cousins all pointed the finger at me, saying I told them it was okay to go. Grandma, who had been watching us, caught us, lined us up, and we received our whippings. She reminded us that there are two roads in life—the right one and the wrong one—and to always choose wisely. At the time, I thought sneaking off was harmless fun, unaware of the dangers in our neighborhood, including drug addicts and gangs. Grandma's lessons on obedience, discernment, and choosing the right path have stayed with me, reflecting the wisdom she instilled from her faith in God. *"The way of fools seems right to them, but the wise listen to advice"* (Proverbs 12:15).

On a cold Saturday morning, I played with Marvin and my cousins flipping over on the mats in our hallway. Then I heard Grandma calling me to her room; she pointed at her chair. I walked over and sat down in the chair. "Tomorrow, we are going to Church. I want you to start learning about the Lord. "Grandma explained the importance of prayer and having God in my life. She told us to say our prayers at night and to always pray. I was so captivated while leaning forward, listening to every word. "You are a good girl. Never change who you are, and never stop learning. Life can be tough, but always work hard and do your best. I had to work hard in my life, but God carried me through some tough times." Grandma told me how challenging it was raising her siblings while taking care of her debilitated mother as a teenager. And after the passing of her mother, she sacrificed her life so they could go to school and have a better life. Raising siblings became a life-changing event in her life, where her role has switched to that of a mother, raising her younger sister and two brothers. I was so intrigued and absorbed every word she said. Sometimes I understood, and some things she shared I couldn't understand. I learned this precious lesson from Grandma about love; we are willing to give anything to ensure our loved ones are safe.

The next day, we all went to church, and I remember enjoying the Sunday school lesson on Noah and the Ark. I was fascinated by God saving Noah, his family, and the animals from the great flood. After the class, I remember sharing what I learned with Grandma while we all walked back home, as I reflected on the importance of prayer and having God in my life. I have always prayed, read the Bible, and kept the hunger and thirst to seek Him throughout my life. And this scripture makes it clear in, *"Those that seek Me early shall find me!"* (Proverbs 8:17). I've learned from Grandma that I'm never alone and have continued an ongoing hunger for Him until my adulthood.

Have you ever been scared for your life? Well, here's an encounter that I will never forget. One hot summer evening, we all just finished seeing a double-feature movie on Times Square and started walking towards the subway, laughing and talking about the film. While walking along, I noticed a bunch of folks standing in a crowd looking at something. Immediately, I was curious to see what the crowd was watching, so I wandered toward the crowd, getting closer and closer to the group. At the same time, I can hear people chattering and a fire truck whisking quickly down the road with sirens fading off into the night. Suddenly, I felt someone gently pulling my left hand backwards; it was very subtle. I assume it was one of my cousins, but it didn't register in my mind, and I had no idea what was happening. With curiosity, I continue to look keenly into the crowd, trying to see among the tall figures in my view.

Then I hear in my spirit a firm voice amidst the noise, crowd, traffic, and chattering among the folks to **turn around and look.** I quickly turned around, looked up, and saw a tall black man beside me.

I was shocked to see this stranger. I frantically snatched my hand, and it slipped away. I began to run so fast while my heart was pounding in my chest until I heard my cousins calling me. I yelled, "Did you see that man?" I heard my cousin say, "What man?" No one saw the man; he vanished quickly. You can believe me when I tell you that I wouldn't be where I am today if God weren't in my life. He's the reason I'm here to tell you my story. I want you to remember whenever you are in a situation or afraid, just remember this scripture:

"Fear not, for I am with you, be not dismayed, for I am your God;
I will strengthen you, I will help you, I will uphold you with my
righteous right hand."
Isaiah 41:10

You can trust His promises in your dire hour to know that God is always right on time. I held on to Grandma's lessons into my adulthood. I carried a burning desire to know Him throughout my career in the military. While stationed at Yokota Air Base in Japan, I always visited the Air Force base chapels and enjoyed the sermons. One Saturday afternoon, I went to a water park with my friends; it would be my last day in Japan. I was delighted to get on the water slide, hugging each curve as it poured me into the pool. I jumped up, filled with enthusiasm, wanting to get on more rides. The next day, I had a piercing, excruciating pain in my left side. After seeing the doctor, he explained to me that it's a pinched nerve. Later, I will learn that relief would come soon when I arrived at my next base in England, United Kingdom.

Upon my arrival, I met Tracey, who welcomed me at the dorm. And she invited me to the base chapel. She introduced me to Jenny and Elaine, still wonderful friends today, after 35 years. Later in the day, I shared with Tracey about the pain in my left side. I was taking Motrin, but when it wore off, the sharp pain came back. On Monday, Tracey told me she had already told the captain, a base chaplain, about the pain I'd been experiencing. She told me to meet with him. At lunchtime, I met with Captain Campbell inside the aircraft hangar, in his trailer. He opened the Bible and read a scripture about healing. Then we prayed together. Captain Campbell asked, "Do you believe?" I said, "Yes."

Later that evening, the pain slowly intensified as the Motrin subsided. I thought about what Grandma had told me–God is always with me and to always pray. I began to pray to God about this pain and believe He would heal me. I heard a pop, and the pain was gone. I got up, thanking God for hearing my prayers and healing me. What a relief! Thank you, Jesus! The pain was gone and never returned. I threw away the Motrin pills. Remember to have faith and trust his promises.

"LORD my God, I called you for help, and you healed me." Psalm 30:2

My grandmother made a lasting impression on my life by sharing her faith in God, which planted the seed in me. I always held on to Grandma's lessons into my adulthood with the burning desire to know Him. I'm grateful and appreciate the importance of her having been in my life. God used my grandmother for His purpose. He knew one day that I would begin my journey in search of Him. God used her for His purpose so that all people would be saved and come to the knowledge of the truth.

"This is good, and pleases God our Savior, who wants all people to be saved and to come to a knowledge of the truth. For there is one God and one mediator between God and mankind, the man Christ Jesus, who gave himself as ransom for all people."
1 Timothy 2:3-6

Notably, here's a powerful story of redemption, a Moabite woman named Ruth. A faithful daughter-in-law to Naomi. Ruth's Israelite husband died before they had a child. She did not return to her mother's house; instead, she stayed with Naomi, her mother-in-law. Ruth turned away from her pagan heritage and followed Naomi back to Bethlehem. She had a gentle and humble heart. She had amazing strength, and she hungered to know about the God of the Israelite people. Even though she was given ample opportunities to stay in her hometown, where things were safe and familiar. She accepted the Lord as her God.

"Look, your sister-in-law has gone back to her people and to her gods. Follow your sister-in-law. But Ruth clung to her mother-in-law. But she replied: don't plead with me to abandon you or return and not follow

you. For wherever you go, I will go, and wherever you live, I will live; your people will be my people, and your God will be my God. Where you die, I will die and there I will be buried. May the Lord punish me, and do so severely, if anything but death separates you and me."
Ruth 1:15-17

Ruth was given permission to glean barley in the field of Boaz, a wealthy relative of Naomi's deceased husband. She diligently works in the fields to provide for herself and Naomi. At the same time, God has embraced Ruth through the actions of Boaz, showing God's willingness to extend redemption to anyone who seeks Him. Ruth listened to Naomi's advice.

"Now isn't Boaz our relative? Haven't you been working with his female servants? This evening, he will be winnowing barley on the threshing floor. Wash on perfumed oil and wear your best clothes. Go down to the threshing floor, but don't let the man know you are there until he has finished eating and drinking. When he lies down, notice the place where he's lying, go in and uncover his feet, and lie down. Then he will explain to you that you should do."
Ruth 3:2-4

When God calls, you must be willing to obey and step out in faith and trust Him, like this story of Ruth pouring out her heart to stay with Naomi. She is willing to sacrifice her life, abandon her pagan customs that have been a part of her entire life, and follow Naomi. God used a widowed woman to serve His purpose. Naomi played a crucial role in guiding Ruth in her interactions with Boaz, and she listened to her. Ruth was a widow during the famine but refused to give up on her husband's people. She devoted herself entirely to Naomi's family and even married Boaz, who was related by marriage to Naomi's husband, Elimelech. Because of this beautiful example of selflessness, she has been honored throughout history.

God had a special plan for Ruth, though she could not have known that she would become part of the tribe of Judah, the great-grandmother of King David, and a key figure in the lineage of Jesus. Her story stands as a timeless example of how faithfulness through difficult times can lead to unexpected blessings. No matter where we are in life or the trials we may face, we can always look to God as our source of strength, trusting that He is weaving a greater purpose for each of us.

Questions:

1. Who has been an influence in your life, and what impact has it made on you?

\
\
\
\
\
\

2. Ruth made a bold move with an act of courage and strength to abandon her culture with grace. What would being bold with grace look like in your own life?

\
\
\
\
\

CHAPTER 3

Lady in Waiting

"Wait for the Lord; be strong and let your heart take courage;
wait for the Lord."
Psalm 27:14

It's a remarkable time to be a woman, living in an era full of opportunities—breaking glass ceilings as pilots, entrepreneurs, business owners, and even running for President. Yet, there is one opportunity often overlooked: the opportunity to wait. Waiting is rarely glamorous. It can feel tedious in a doctor's office or while on hold listening to, 'You are number ten in line, please wait.' But there's a deeper, more challenging kind of waiting—the kind that tests your patience and faith: waiting for a job call, medical results, or the right partner.

I know this personally. In my thirties, unmarried and feeling the pressure of my biological clock, I faced the challenges of dating, seeking someone whose values aligned with God. I prayed for a husband using 'The List,' detailing the qualities I desired in a future spouse. A friend, Sonya, encouraged me to try the newspaper classifieds—back then, before online dating was common. That led me to meet Greg, and two years later, we married, and I was at the age of thirty-six.

Though Greg has passed on to glory, I remain deeply grateful for the time we shared. During our courtship, we attended church together, prayed, and read the Bible. I introduced him to my brother and sister in Christ, William and Leola Simmons, a couple devoted to the Lord. We had Bible study every Tuesday at their home, filled with delicious food, fellowship, and love. At the time, he was Catholic, seeking more about Christ, and studying the Word enlightened him. He decided he wanted to get baptized that night after reading: *"For there is one God and one mediator between God and mankind, the man Christ Jesus, who gave himself as a ransom for all people*" (1 Timothy 2:5-6). We all went to the church building, and Bro Simmons baptized him. Also, Sis Simmons did the catering and baked a beautiful wedding cake for our Wedding. Both have passed on to glory, and I will forever cherish them in my heart. Looking back, I see that the season of waiting—though challenging—brought lessons and blessings far beyond what I could have imagined, shaping my faith, patience, and appreciation for God's timing.

As a matter of fact, there's no set formula for how life should unfold. We simply need to walk our journey with the Lord and trust His timing. When we know that God is the Author of our story, we can find peace in knowing He is guiding us toward good things. God desires a deep, personal relationship with us, and times of waiting often draw us closer to Him, teaching us patience and dependence. In the end, His timing ensures we receive His very best.

In this season of singleness, remember there is always hope. Jesus is not finished writing your story, and if it isn't good yet, it simply means He's still at work. God knows you intimately—every detail of your life—and you are precious to Him. You have captured His heart and His full attention. Here's comfort in knowing Psalm 139

You have searched me, LORD, and you know me.
You know when I sit and when I rise; you perceive my thoughts from afar.
You discern my going out and my lying down; you are familiar with all my ways.
Before a word is on my tongue you, LORD, know it completely.
You hem me in behind and before, and you lay your hand upon me.
Such knowledge is too wonderful for me, too lofty for me to attain.
Where can I go from your Spirit? Where can I flee from your presence?
If I go up to the heavens, you are there; if I make my bed in the depths, you are there.
If I rise on the wings of the dawn, if I settle on the far side of the sea,
Even there your hand will guide me, your right hand will hold me fast.

If I say, "Surely the darkness will hide me and the light become night around me,"
Even the darkness will not be dark to you; the night will shine like the day, for darkness
is as light to you
For you created my inmost being; you knit me together in my mother's womb.
I praise you because I am fearfully and wonderfully made; your works are wonderful; I know that full well.
My frame was not hidden from you when I was made in the secret place, when I was woven together in the depths of the earth.
Your eyes saw my uniformed body; all the days ordained for me were written in your book before one of them came to be.
How precious to me are your thoughts, God! How vast is the sum of them!
Were I to count them, they would outnumber the grains of sand; when I awake, I am still with you.
If only you, God, would slay the wicked! Away from me, you who are bloodthirsty!
They speak of you with evil intent; your adversaries misuse your name.
Do I not hate those who hate you, LORD, and abhor those who are in rebellion again you?
I have nothing but hatred for them; I count them my enemies.
Search me, God, and know my heart; test me and know my anxious thoughts
See if there is any offensive way in me, and lead me in the way everlasting.

For this reason, do not feel you are singled out in a coupled world. Being single can be a blessing because you can walk in the fullness of who God called you to be, regardless of your status. I want to encourage you to know that Jesus loves you! You are blessed, and He knows everything about you! He is with you always, and will never leave nor forsake you. Let's remember that this season is a time for personal growth, self-sufficiency, and preparation for the future. It's an opportunity to pursue your goals while trusting God's perfect timing for your life. One of the greatest lies of the enemy is convincing you that you are running out of time—but with God, His timing is always right on schedule.

Still, there is something special in a season of waiting, namely, a woman who waits on the Lord. In fact, biblical history has been significantly marked by them. According to the scriptures, the word "wait" normally suggests the anxious, yet confident, expectation by God's people that the Lord will intervene on their behalf. Such waiting may be for answers to prayers (Psalms 25:5), for the coming of the Holy Spirit (Acts 1:4), for salvation (Genesis 49:18), or especially for the coming of the Messiah to bring salvation to His people and establish His Kingdom on earth (Psalms 37:35; Luke 12:36; Romans 8:23; 1 Thessalonians 1:10).

Likewise, here's a faithful and praying woman named Hannah, who was unable to bear children. She suffered ridicule from Elkanah's other wife, Peninnah, who bore him several children. Not to mention, Hannah ached for a child of her own, and this is during a culture that saw the blessing of children as the greatest possible good and a sign of God's favor. Just imagine, Hannah must have felt like being shut out of God's grace. And it was especially painful to be compared to other women who not only had children of their own, but also turned that beautiful gift into a weapon by mocking and belittling childless women. Reading this story, Hannah would have likely felt depressed, as though her life was meaningless, and was insulted daily by dealing with her infertility. She was so brokenhearted that she couldn't receive her husband's kindness, eat her food, or stop weeping.

"Whenever Elkanah offered a sacrifice, he always gave portions of the meat to his wife Peninnah and to each of her sons and daughters. But he gave a double portion to Hannah, for he loved her even though the Lord had kept her from conceiving. Her rival would taunt her severely just to provoke her, because the Lord had kept Hannah from conceiving. Year after year, when she went up to the Lord's house, her rival taunted her in this way. Hannah would weep and would not eat."
- 1 Samuel 4-8.

Imagine the pain of sharing a spouse with another wife who had many children—Hannah must have felt isolated and deeply hurt. In response to her broken heart, she went to the Lord's house to pray, pouring out her soul and weeping bitterly. Her grief was so intense that Eli, the priest, thought she was drunk. Hannah vowed that if God gave her a son, she would dedicate him to the Lord's service. God answered her prayers, and she gave birth to the prophet Samuel, faithfully fulfilling her promise. Though Elkanah was married to two women, he loved Hannah deeply, much like Jacob loved Rachel, and he recognized her suffering.

"Please my lord," she said, "as surely as you live, my lord, I am the woman who stood here beside you praying to the Lord. I prayed for this boy, and since the Lord gave me what I asked him for. I now give the boy to the Lord. For as long as he lives, he is given to the Lord." Then he worshipped the Lord there." 1 Samuel 1:26-28

We can learn from Hannah, no matter what challenges or desires we may have, to go to God. We can do what Hannah did! You may not think of yourself as the most spiritual person or strong in your faith, especially when you compare yourself to other women, but what's so remarkable about Hannah was that she prayed to God and He extended grace to her. Hannah sought the Lord alone for her heart's desires, and she kept her promise to the Lord, giving her son to Eli with thanksgiving and joy. Your waiting is not in vain. Here's what's so interesting to me. Hannah wanted a son, but God wanted a prophet for Israel. God had to bring Hannah to the point of desperation so that she was not only crying out to the Lord for a child but was willing to give her child up for the Lord's service. She wanted a son, but God needed a prophet. God had to bring Hannah to the place where she wanted what God wanted. God doesn't promise that things are going to be easy, but He does promise us victory if we don't give up.

"What then are we to say about these things?
If God is for us, who is against us?"
Romans 8:31

Equally important, we meet Anna, a prophetess, who spent all her days at the temple for the Messiah. Both Hannah's and Anna's names mean grace, and they show us how to trust God in our waiting season. Anna proclaimed the love of God to anyone who stood long enough to listen to her. She was a widow, daughter of Phanuel of the tribe of Asher. She was at the temple in Jerusalem when Mary and Joseph brought Jesus to be dedicated. Anna recognized Jesus as the long-awaited Messiah.

"Anna was a widow for eighty-four years. She did not leave the temple, serving God night and day with fasting and prayers. At that very moment, she came up and began to thank God and to speak about him to all who were looking forward to the redemption of Jerusalem. When they had completed everything according to the law of the Lord, they returned to Galilee, to their own town of Nazareth. The boy grew up and became strong, filled with wisdom and God's grace was on Him."
Luke 2:37-40

We can learn so much from the way God rewarded Anna's faith, obedience, and expectancy. Anna dedicated her life to dwelling in the temple of the Lord, spending the rest of her years fasting, in prayer, and worship. She could have easily remarried and started a new life. Yet, her ultimate choice was to remain in the temple in anticipation of the Messiah. She arrived at the moment Simeon was blessing baby Jesus and prophesying about Him. She recognized the Christ child and began praising God.

Anna waited a long time, walking in obedience for Jesus. She kept telling others about the redemption of Israel that God would be sending soon. Sometimes we may get discouraged in our walk of faith or ministry, but Anna teaches us to persevere. She inspires us to tell everyone we meet about our wonderful Savior, Jesus Christ. She showed us that touching lives with the truth holds a great reward, especially when you see the transformation of those hearts that lead to redemption. She teaches us that God can use anyone. We may look at our lives and think what God could possibly want to use us for, but he draws us out of our comfort zone to serve His purpose. God gets the glory. Always remember, God's perfect timing is found when you are sensitive to His Spirit and follow His prompting.

Questions:

1. How did Hannah demonstrate her faith? And what has her story taught you when faced with life challenges?

____

____

____

____

____

2. Anna spent her final days on earth sharing the gospel about Christ. How will you spend your life?

____

____

____

____

____

CHAPTER 4

God's Grace

*"The grace of the Lord Jesus Christ, and the love of God, and the
fellowship of the Holy Spirit be with you all."*
2 Corinthians 13:13

Grace! Can we earn it or work for it? No. God is gracious. Because of His love, God, who is rich in mercy, saved us by grace. The grace of God was supremely revealed and given in the person and work of Jesus Christ. Jesus restored the broken fellowship between God and His people through His death and resurrection.

*"Therefore, if anyone is in Christ, he is a new creation; the old has
passed away, and see, the new has come! Everything is from God,
who has reconciled us to himself through Christ and has given us the
ministry of reconciliation. That is, in Christ, God was reconciling the
world to himself, not counting their trespasses against them, and he
has committed the message of reconciliation to us. Therefore, we are
ambassadors for Christ, since God is making his appeal through us. We
plead on Christ's behalf. "Be reconciled to God." He made the one who
did not know sin to be sin for us, so that in Him
we might become the righteousness of God."*
2 Corinthians 5:17-22

Can God bring people into your life for a reason? I'm here to tell you, He does. In the fall of 1993, while stationed at Dyess Air Force Base in Abilene, Texas, I separated and moved to Dallas, Texas. I asked my Air Force buddy and roommate, Sonya Jones, a native Texan, about finding a church home. Another wonderful friend, Sonya, and I were stationed at my first base at Yokota Air Base, Japan, in 1987. We were searching for a church home and visited many churches in the DFW metroplex. She told me her brother, Bobby, goes to a church named Greenville Avenue Church of Christ in Richardson, and we are both still members today.

In 1995, I moved to Arlington to attend college, still searching for a church home. I asked God to help me find a church home where I could grow and learn His word. One afternoon, I went to Office Max to type a letter for school on one of the Brother electric typewriters. I walked over to the copier machine to make a copy. Then I see a white paper with handwritten words: Out of Service. The only available one had a lady standing over it, photocopying a page from the textbook. I stood behind her, waiting impatiently. I asked, "Are you going to make all those copies?"

As a matter of fact, the woman's name is Sherry, and we began talking about school and the Lord. She asked me if I had a church home. I explained to her about not finding a church home, but I like the powerful sermon the preacher gave at the church I visited in Richardson, with Sonya. Surprisingly, Sherry tells me she attends Sherman Street Church of Christ in Grand Prairie. And she invited me to her home and shared with me about the Bible and getting baptized. Later that evening, I read the passage from the Book of Acts about how Peter tells the house of Israel that God has made Jesus, who was crucified and resurrected as both Lord and Christ. I read Acts 2:36-42 and thanked Jesus for answering my prayer.

"Therefore, let all the house of Israel know with certainty that God has made this Jesus, whom your crucified, both Lord and Messiah." When they heard this, they were pierced to the heart and said to Peter and the rest of the apostles: Brothers, what should we do?" Peter replied. "Repent and be baptized, each of you in the name of Jesus Christ for the forgiveness of your sins, and you will receive the gift of the Holy Spirit. For the promise is for you and for your children, and for all who are far off, as many as the Lord our God will call. With many other words he testified and strongly urged them, saying, "Be saved from this corrupt generation!" So those who accepted this message were baptized, and that day about three thousand people were added to them. They devoted themselves to the apostles teaching, to the fellowship, to the breaking of bread, and to prayer.

The following Sunday, I went to church with Sherry Ann Brown. I went down the aisle, got baptized, and began my journey as a new convert. This is grace! God showed me grace and mercy by washing away my sins. Being baptized into Christ means identifying with Him in His death, burial, and resurrection. We died with Him, and through Him, received a new life in which we are set free from sin. This means our old sinful selves were crucified with Christ so that sin might lose its power in our lives. We are no longer slaves to sin. For when we died with Christ, we were set free from the power of sin.

"For we know that our old self was crucified with Him so that the body ruled by sin might be rendered powerless so that we may no longer be enslaved to sin. Since a person who has died is freed from sin."
Romans 6:6-7

One night while I was lying in bed, I heard His voice. "Finally, you come to Me." **I will never forget the moment when Jesus wrapped His loving arms around me, filling me with an overwhelming abundance of love and peace—words could never fully capture the richness of what I felt.**

I share this lesson because my grandmother planted the seed of faith in me, a seed that profoundly shaped my life and ultimately led me to Christ. Though she could not read, her wisdom was boundless, and she taught me the importance of keeping God at the center of everything I do. I carried that lesson into adulthood, holding it close through every challenge and decision. Guided by faith, I took a bold step and left Brooklyn, New York, to join the Air Force, trusting that God would lead the way.

Despite initially failing the Armed Services Vocational Aptitude Battery (ASVAB), I joined the Air Force after persistent studying and practice with a Marine recruiter. One freezing day, I went to the recruiting station to practice and noticed a note on the door: "Due to a family emergency, I'm rescheduling for next Saturday." I decided to stay and warm my hands before heading back outside; it was freezing with snow on the ground. I walked down the hall, passing the Army office—no one was inside—and then the Navy office, which was also empty.

At the end of the hall, I looked to my left and saw inside the sky-blue painted office, where the words "Aim High" were painted on the wall. The recruiter was sitting at his desk, wearing a light blue pressed shirt and dark navy-blue pants, with multicolored ribbons pinned centered on the left side of his shirt.

He asked me, "Can I help you?"
I replied, "No, I'm just warming my hands."
He asked if I had heard of the Air Force, and I said, "No, I haven't."
He then told me, "Come on in and sit down."
He asked if I had taken the ASVAB standardized test. I explained that I had taken it but didn't pass, which is why I was there practicing.
He said, "Well, if you've been practicing, I think you should be ready to take the exam."

As a result, I took the test, passed, and received a departure date for the following year to begin six weeks of basic training at Lackland Air Force Base in San Antonio, Texas.

In the meantime, I needed to go to Fort Hamilton to complete my physical exam and get sworn in. In fact, I'm grateful for the opportunity to serve in the Air Force; the challenges and training have allowed me to travel overseas. Meeting new people has made a huge impact on my life. I also enjoyed volunteering. Being a Big Sister to three Little Sisters was very rewarding, and one is now in college. I stay active in my church, and being involved in the prison ministry is a great way to participate in God's work. I have learned to trust God and realize that He always shows me grace and mercy, guiding my path to Him.

As for you, reader, do you know your purpose in life? In the Bible, it says, "For I know the plans I have for you, "declares the Lord, plans to prosper you and not harm you, plans to give you hope and a future" (Jeremiah 29:11).

As a matter of fact, here's the story of a courageous woman, where leadership can come from unexpected places. Rahab was a Canaanite and a prostitute who lived in Jericho; she was not valued by her people. Like Ruth, Rahab left her culture of worshipping many gods of her ancestors to follow the one true God, unlike Timothy, who had a grandmother, Eunice, and Mother Lois, who diligently nurtured their children in the faith and understood the importance of teaching children God's Word at a young age. Yet, Rahab showed the fruit of her faith.

"You see that a person is justified by works and not by faith alone. In the same way, wasn't Rahab the prostitute also justified by works in receiving the messengers and sending them out by a different route? For just as the body without the spirit is dead, so also faith without works is dead."
James 2:24-26

Rahab's house was built in the wall, and Joshua sent a couple of spies ahead of his army to scout the land. She hid two Israelite spies, helping them to escape, and stood against the king of Jericho. She covered them with stalks of flax and told them where to go and how long they should hide. She planned the protection and the escape of the two spies through a window using a heavy scarlet rope.

Joshua son of Nun secretly sent two men as spies from the Acacia Grove, saying, "Go and scout the land, especially Jericho." So, they left, and they came to the house of a prostitute named Rahab and stayed there. The King of Jericho was told, "Look, some of the Israelite men have come here tonight to investigate the land." Then the King of Jericho sent word to Rahab and said, "Bring out the men who came to you and entered your house, for they came to investigate the entire land."
Joshua 2:1-3

Somehow, news spread of the Hebrew visitors, and the king ordered Rahab to give them up. However, Rahab was courageous, and her faith in God's power and her actions demonstrate the importance of acting on one's faith. Rahab had heard about how God saved Israel and dried up the Red Sea.

"For we have heard how the Lord dried up the water of the Red Sea before you when you came out of Egypt, and what you did to Sihon and Og, the two Amorite Kings you completely destroyed across the Jordan.

*When we heard this, we lost heart, and everyone's courage failed
because of you for the Lord your God is God in heaven above and on
Earth below."
Joshua 2:10-11*

When the Israelites captured Jericho, they paired the house with the scarlet cord in the window, a sign that a friend of God's people lived within. Rahab, therefore, along with her father, her mother, her brothers, and her father's household, was spared. Rahab made bold decisions to place themselves at risk for the sake of God's people. As a matter of fact, Rahab was adopted as one of God's own and became part of the bloodline of the royal family. She was the wife of Salmon, and their son Boaz married Ruth. This amazing story of a Canaanite harlot became part of the lineage of King David, out of which the Messiah came. God showed Rahab's grace, and she risked her life for His people. She reminds us that we can take risks for God, no matter what the circumstances may be. Just trust Him. Rahab chose to trust and obey the One and True God!

On the other hand, we have a woman with the reputation for being a "sinner" who had heard of Jesus' arrival. She approached Jesus at Simon's home, bringing a jar of perfume with which to anoint Him. She washed His feet with her tears, wiping them with her hair and anointing them with the perfume.

*"Then one of the Pharisees invited Him to eat with him. He entered the
Pharisee's house and reclined at the table. And a woman in the town
who was a sinner found out that Jesus was reclining at the table in the
Pharisee's house. She brought an alabaster jar of perfume, and stood
behind him at his feet, weeping, and began to wash his feet with her
tears. She wiped His feet with her hair, kissing them and anointing
them with the perfume."
Luke 7:36-38*

Regardless, Simon recoils from the woman's generosity and shows no hesitation in describing the woman as a sinner. She was undesirable and would never have been welcome in the home of a well-respected Pharisee.

"When the Pharisee who had invited Him saw this, he said to himself, 'This man, if He were a prophet, would know who and what kind of woman this is who is touching Him, she's a sinner!"
Luke 7:39

Still, the woman never spoke, but her tears flowed as she poured out her heart in extravagant worship.

Jesus replied to him, "Simon, I have something to say to you." He said, "Say it teacher." A creditor had two debtors. One owed five hundred denarii, and the other fifty. Since they could not pay it back, he graciously forgave them both. So, which of them will love him more?" Simon answered, "I suppose the one he forgave more." "You have judged correctly, he told Him. "Turning to the woman, he said to Simon, "Do you see this woman? I entered your house; you gave me no water for my feet, but she, with her tears, has washed my feet and wiped them with her hair. You gave me no kiss, but she hasn't stopped kissing my feet since I came in. You didn't anoint my head with olive oil, but she has anointed my feet with perfume. Therefore, I tell you, her many sins have been forgiven; that's why she loves much. But the one who is forgiven little, loves little. Then He said to her, "Your sins are forgiven."
Luke 7:40-48

Indeed, Jesus's ministry to the sinful woman beautifully demonstrates the fulfillment of Isaiah's prophecy (Isaiah 52:7). A Pharisee, who was quite learned in the Word of God, did not recognize this truth. However, a sinful woman, an outcast, acknowledged the prophecy and demonstrated her understanding of it by focusing on the feet of the greatest Prophet, the One destined to bring her peace and salvation.

And He said to the woman. "Your faith has saved you. Go in peace."
Luke 7:50

Like Rahab, we can see this woman was not valued among the people; she was an outcast; however, she was persistent with her generosity to Jesus. While he was busy condemning the sinful woman, he failed the basic test of hospitality. Who was the greater sinner, the woman who worshiped Jesus extravagantly, or the self-righteous attitude of the Pharisee Simon, who not only lacked true understanding of his own need for forgiveness but also refused to show generosity in worship? This story has so many lessons to teach us about God's abundant forgiveness, the depth of true repentance, and recognizing one's need for God's grace.

In addition, I welcome you to apply these lessons and examine your heart, reflect on your own motivations, and consider whether your actions stem from genuine repentance and love for God, and not just outward appearances. Most importantly, show gratitude, extend compassion, and understand those who may be struggling with sin, just as Jesus did for the sinful woman, who became a forgiven sinner.

Questions:

1. How did Hannah demonstrate her faith? And what has her story taught you when faced with life challenges?

____

55

____

____

____

____

2. Anna spent her final days on earth sharing the gospel about Christ. How will you spend your life?

____

____

____

____

____

CHAPTER 5

Speak Wisely

"Do not let any unwholesome talk come out of your mouths, but only what is helpful for building others up according to their needs, that it may benefit those who listen."
Ephesians 4:29

We may have heard the classic warning, "Be careful of what you say to people". Maybe we struggle with fear or anger or bitterness, or maybe our words are hopeful or encouraging or thoughtful. The bottom line is we need to choose our words wisely and to start by looking at our hearts and examining them.

"A good person produces good out of the good stored up in his heart. An evil person produces evil stored in his heart, for his mouth speaks from the overflow of the heart."
Luke 6:45

Just think about it! Our words impact us and those around us every single day. This means we face a choice: how do we want to use our words? We can choose to speak wisely or be confrontational to get our point across. One evening, I was typing my 10-page term paper due the next day. I heard loud music coming from the apartment above me. My neighbor was playing loud heavy metal music turned all the way up. I could hear the roaring bass shake the walls, and at this point, I couldn't concentrate on my paper. I walked upstairs and knocked on his door, where a short Caucasian man opened it. I politely asked if he could turn his music down because it was shaking the walls in my apartment. He apologized and turned his music down.

A few weeks later, I was taking a nap before starting my 11 pm -7 am shift. I heard my neighbor upstairs barking like a dog: Woof! Woof! Woof! He continued to bark loudly out his window. At the time, I had a cocker spaniel with me, and he wasn't barking. I couldn't sleep with my neighbor barking and howling like a dog repeatedly. So, I decided not to go upstairs to confront him; instead, I called the police about the barking. When two officers arrived, they saw my neighbor in the bushes near my patio. I was peering through my blinds, trying to see what he was doing in the bushes. One of the officers asked, "Hey, what are you looking for?" He looked up and replied, "I was yelling out my window, and my teeth fell out. I'm trying to find my teeth."

One morning, I was walking to my apartment after working the night shift when I saw the maintenance guy cleaning out my neighbor's apartment. I asked him what was going on. He explained that there had been a lot of complaints from the tenants about this guy, so he's not going to be living there anymore. I looked around and saw the man had trashed his apartment; it was filled with holes in the walls and inflated dolls on the floor. It was a mess. I was also surprised when he told me there had been numerous complaints from other neighbors behind and beside his apartment. I thought it was just me calling in the complaints. I looked around his apartment with a big sigh of relief.

> *"The one who guards his mouth and tongue*
> *keeps himself out of trouble."*
> *Proverbs 21-23*

How do you respond when you need to have a difficult conversation with someone you love? Here's a warm story about Abigail, a beautiful, godly woman who earned a good reputation as a peacemaker. She was a woman of wisdom, discernment, a sharp mind, and a generous spirit who always treated people with respect, even in tough circumstances.

Abigail was married to a very wealthy man named Nabal, who had large flocks of sheep. However, he was foolish, ill-tempered, and drunken, and she had dealt with an unhappy marriage by conducting herself with respect and avoiding confrontation with her husband, while speaking persuasively. Also, it was customary at sheep-shearing time for the master to host a celebration for his household and servants, and Nabal had made festive preparations for them. Meanwhile, Nabal's men were shearing his sheep, while David's men provided protection for their flocks as they traveled through the region. David sent his men to ask Nabal to show favor to them by sharing some of their provisions.

Instead, Nabal, being the harsh, headstrong man he was, responded to David's request with insults.

"David's young men went and said all these things to Nabal on David's
behalf, and they waited. Nabal asked them, "Who is David? Who
is Jesse's son? Many slaves these days are running away from their
masters. Am I supposed to take my bread, my water, and my meat that
I butchered for my shearers and give them to these men? I don't know
where they are from." David's young men retraced their steps. When
they returned to him, they reported all these words. He said to his men.
"All of you put on your swords!" So each man put on his sword, and
David also put on his sword. About four hundred men followed David
while two hundred stayed with the supplies. One of Nabal's young men
informed Abigail, Nabal's wife: "Look, David sent messengers from
the wilderness to greet our master, but he screamed at them. The men
treated us very well. When we were in the field, we weren't harassed,
and nothing of ours was missing the whole time we were living among
them. They were a wall around us, both day and night, the entire time
we were with them, herding the sheep. Now consider carefully what you
should do, because there is certain to be trouble for our master and his
entire family. He is such a worthless fool, nobody can talk to him!"
1 Samuel 25:9-16

Also, the servants talked with Abigail when they were afraid to talk to Nabal. A servant's life in his household was never pleasant, and it suddenly turned catastrophic when Nabal insulted David, the future King of Israel. Now, with the lives of Nabal and his servants hanging in the balance. Well, here you see the dilemma of Abigail. She is caught between a fool and a King who is acting like a fool. What is she to do? David has set out to kill her husband. God also planned to use Abigail to protect His king from doing something very foolish and costly. Yet God was also using Abigail to protect her own husband from a savage death. This is all about God! God gave Abigail the wisdom to know what to do in the instant a decision had to be made. No matter how you are threatened and no matter how you are pushed to decide, God will answer you! He will use you to accomplish His divine plan.

Abigail, in her wisdom, gathered enough food for David's men, rode out to meet David, and bowed before him to show her respect. By agreeing with David that Nabal had acted with great disrespect, she calmed David's anger. Abigail's quick action of speaking wisely and respectfully averted the disaster. In this case, no one really enjoys conflict. If possible, most of us prefer to avoid confrontations. The world around us is filled with tension, with constant news of war and political unrest, all we want is a little peace and quiet, that's it! When our relationships feel strained, we immediately turn the other way, bury our heads in the sand, and hope it all goes away. Yet, when conflict arose between Nabal and David, Abigail did not run from the situation. In fact, she used many of her gifts to calm the chaos. Abigail acted to protect two men who had grown hotheaded and argumentative. She refused to sit by passively and let the conflict escalate; instead, she chose to confront it.

"As she rode the donkey down a mountain pass hidden from view, she saw David and his men coming toward her and met them. David had just said, "I guarded everything that belonged to this man in the wilderness for nothing. He was not missing anything, yet he paid me back evil for good. May God punish me and do so severely if I let any of his males survive until morning. When Abigail saw David, she quickly got off the donkey and knelt down with her face to the ground and paid homage to David. She knelt at his feet and said, "The guilt is mine, my lord, but please let your servant speak to you directly. Listen to the words of your servant. My lord should pay no attention to this worthless fool, Nabal, for he lives up to his name. His name means stupid, and stupidity is all he knows. I, your servant, didn't see my lord's young men whom you sent. Now my lord, as surely as the Lord lives and as you yourself live, it is the Lord who kept you from participating in bloodshed and avenging yourself by your own hand. May your enemies and those who intend to harm my lord be like Nabal. Let this gift your servant has brought to my lord be given to the young men who follow my lord. Please forgive your servant's offense, for the Lord is certain to make a lasting dynasty for my lord because he fights the Lord's battles. Throughout your life, may evil not be found to you."
1 Samuel 25:20-28

It's important to recognize that David not only feels that Nabal has insulted him but also that Nabal has insulted God. Therefore, David asks God to give him the strength to bring justice against Nabal. Isn't it remarkable how, when we are hurt, we often think we have the right to respond, sometimes even more harshly than the person who offended us? Of course, Nabal was wrong, but so was David. As you can see, God had a purpose for Abigail, and she recognized how foolish Nabal was, and it seems she understood how reckless David was acting. Yet she took responsibility for the entire conflict and bore the blame herself, hoping David would not take out his anger on her. Another key point is that Abigail did not get angry or lose her temper; instead, she calmly persuaded David to let his enemies look like fools, but urged him not to behave like one because he's the King. Wow! This demonstrates incredible discernment. Abigail was clearly guided by God, showing wisdom that could only come from divine insight. Eventually, Abigail told Nabal about her meeting with David, and he became very upset, to the point of illness.

"Then Abigail went to Nabal, and there he was in his house, holding a feast fit for a king. Nabal's heart was cheerful, and he was very drunk, so she didn't say anything to him until morning light. In the morning when Nabal sobered up, his wife told him about these events. His heart died and he became a stone. About ten days later, the Lord struck Nabal dead."
1 Samuel 25:36-38

We can learn many lessons from Abigail; she demonstrated self-control when dealing with difficult people and situations. Abigail's actions showed her wise and godly heart. She never got angry, lost her temper, nagged her husband, called him a fool, or complained about how many times she told him to do something despite his temper. Abigail had faith in God and recognized His plan for Israel regarding David. She possessed wisdom, forgiveness, good judgment, and made wise decisions. In a surprising turn of events, after Nabal died of a heart attack ten days later, David took Abigail as his wife. God rewarded Abigail's gracious conduct by freeing her from Nabal and blessing her with a happier future.

As for you, reader, you may not be facing a specific enemy right now, but Abigail's story clearly shows that crises do not define character; they reveal it. She also demonstrated that humility, honor, and respect have the power to defeat your enemies and even inspire their agreement with you.

Questions:

1. How do you respond when you need to have a difficult conversation with someone you love? And what are some practical ways we can negotiate and become a peacemaker in conflict situations?

63

____

____

____

____

____

2. What is one conflicted situation you are facing in this season of your life?

____

____

____

____

____

CHAPTER 6

A Faithful Witness

"But in your hearts revere Christ as Lord. Always be prepared to give an answer to everyone who ask you to give the reason for the hope that you have. But do this with gentleness and respect,"
1 Peter 3:15-16

Maybe you're afraid to share your faith because you don't know what to say, or maybe you're sharing the Gospel, but nothing is happening; people aren't committing their lives to Christ. Are you doing something wrong? Jesus demonstrated a remarkable ability to meet people in their mess and to accept them and love them as they were without condoning their lifestyles.

"Indeed, we have all received grace upon grace from His fullness, for the law was given through Moses; grace and truth came through Jesus Christ. No one has ever seen God. The one and only Son, who is himself God and is at the Father's side, He has revealed Him."
John 1:16-18

Even though we live in a broken world, surrounded by broken lives and relationships, this brokenness is evident in the suffering, violence, poverty, pain, and death all around us. However, it can lead us to seek ways to make life work. You can also share your faith with people in your life—family, friends, neighbors, and co-workers—and pray to God to guide someone into your life who needs Him. In fact, I once had a screensaver on my work computer that showed flying windows. Back in the day, these screensavers appeared after a few minutes to prevent burn-in, but we still use them today because they're entertaining and interesting to look at.

Then one day, I decided to change my screensaver to Winnie the Pooh with the scriptures. A coworker walked by my desk, and she saw my new screensaver flashing vibrant colors of Winnie the Pooh dancing, holding a jar of honey, in the park while the red, orange, and yellow leaves floated down with the scriptures displaying: "Gracious words are a honeycomb, sweet to the soul and health to the bones" (Proverbs 16:24). She stopped at my desk and told me she liked my screensaver. She asked me if I could put this on her computer. I said, "Sure." Surprisingly, this was the beginning of a new friendship—she was looking for a church home. I was glad to share with her about my church, where we have great Bible study classes, and I invited her to our Ladies Symposium that was coming up in a week. Later, after she attended the Bible study classes, she got baptized, and we are still friends today. After 23 years, Daphne still loves to talk about the stories in the Bible, and we often discuss biblical characters and which book of the Bible we are studying.

At the same time, we must do more than live godly lives; people are searching and need to hear the Gospel, to hear that God loves them. Christ died for them so that they can have eternal life.

"How, then, can they call on Him they have not believed in? And how can they believe without hearing about him? And how can they hear without a preacher? And how they preach unless they are sent? As it is written: How beautiful are the feet of those who bring good news. But not all obeyed the gospel. For Isaiah says, Lord, who has believed our message? So, faith come from what is heard, and what is heard comes through the message about Christ."
Romans 10:14-17

Like the story in the Bible about the conversion of the Ethiopian who was reading the book of Isaiah while traveling in a chariot but was perplexed by the passage, Philip, one of Jesus's 12 disciples, was guided by an angel to help the high-ranking Ethiopian court official.

"An angel of the Lord spoke to Philip: 'Get up and go south to the road that goes down from Jerusalem to Gaza." So, he got up and went. There was an Ethiopian man, a eunuch and high official of Candace, queen of the Ethiopians, who was in charge of her entire treasury. He had come to worship in Jerusalem and was sitting in his chariot on his way home, reading the prophet Isaiah aloud. The Spirit told Philip, "Go and

join that chariot." When Philip ran up to it, he heard him reading the prophet Isaiah, and said, "Do you understand what you're reading?" "How can I," he said, "unless someone guides me?" So, he invited Philip to come up and sit with him. Now the scripture passage he was reading was this: He was led like a sheep to the slaughter, and as a lamb is silent before its shearer, so he does not open his mouth. In humiliation, justice was denied him. Who will describe His generation? For His life is taken from the earth. The eunuch said to Philip, "I ask you, who is this prophet saying this about himself or someone else? Philip proceeded to tell him the good news about Jesus, beginning with that Scripture. As they were traveling down the road, they came to some water. The eunuch said, "Look, there's water. What would keep me from being baptized?" So, he ordered the chariot to stop, and both Philip and the eunuch went down into the water, and he baptized him. When they came up out of the water, the Spirit of the Lord carried Philip away, and the eunuch did not see him any longer but went on his way rejoicing."
Acts 8:26-39

When we next meet a faithful witness, a young, courageous Hebrew girl who had been captured and brought to Syria. She is a servant to the wife of Naaman, commander of the Syrian army, serving as her maidservant. Her place in history is brief and not even marked by her name. While Naaman was a highly regarded military commander, he suffered from leprosy, which was incurable and made Naaman a societal outcast. Naaman's maidservant was taken to Syria during the reign of Ahab's son, Joram. Ahab was married to Jezebel. This was a time when surrounding nations constantly invaded Israel, and the maidservant was living in a foreign land, serving people who may have killed her family. Despite the oppression of war, this young girl was determined to reveal the superiority of Israel's God over the pagan gods of Syria. She exercised her simple faith and testified to God's power to heal.

"Naaman, commander of the army for the king of Aram, was a man important to his master and highly regarded because through him, the Lord had given victory to Aram. The man was a valiant warrior, but he had a skin disease. Aram had gone on raids and brought back from the land of Israel a young girl who served Naaman's wife. She said to her mistress, "If only my master were with the prophet who is in Samaria,

he would cure him of his skin disease. So Naaman went and told his master what the girl from the land of Israel had said. Therefore, the king of Aram said, "Go, and I will send a letter with you to the King of Israel." So, he went and took 750 pounds of silver, 150 pounds of gold, and ten sets of clothing. He brought the letter to the King of Israel, and it read: When this letter comes to you, note that I have sent you my servant Naaman for you to cure him of his skin disease."
2 Kings 5:1-6

It is important to realize that this Hebrew child had clearly been taught that God's hand was on her life. Even though she was in a pagan environment, she remained firmly committed to Yahweh as a God of mercy. She bravely exercised her faith, which led not only to the miracle of saving her master's life but also to his introduction to the power of the God of Israel. Her persistent testimony caused Naaman to set aside his pride and decide to put his faith in the God of Israel.

"So Naaman went down and dipped himself in the Jordan seven times, according to the command of the man of God. Then his skin was restored and became like skin of small boy and he was clean. The Naaman and his whole company went back to the man of God, stood before him, and declared. "I know there's no God in the whole world except in Israel. Therefore, please accept a gift from your servant." But Elisha said, "As the Lord lives, in whose presence I stand, I will not accept it." Naaman urged him to accept it, but he refused."
2 Kings 5:14-16

As for you, reader, there are lessons from Naaman's maidservant. She shares her faith with her captor even though she could have kept quiet. This child's simple faith, her confidence in God's prophet, Elisha, and her desire for her master's welfare led to Naaman's miraculous healing. She was an instrument of God even in a difficult circumstance. Her actions changed Naaman's life forever, and he became a worshiper of God. Also, have a positive attitude and show God's love to others. Like the servant girl reflected God's love to her captors, even though they were enemies. Despite dire situations, take advantage of opportunities to serve; like the servant girl, she acted immediately when her opportunity to serve the Lord arose. Most of all, stand on your faith; it takes courage, and don't be afraid to do the right thing.

Questions:

1. What did Naaman's maidservant do?

2. Why was this courageous? And how can we apply this lesson to our lives?

CHAPTER 7

A Listening Heart

"Pay attention and turn your ear to the sayings of the wise; apply your heart to what I teach, for it is pleasing when you keep them in your heart and have all of them ready on your lips."
Proverbs 22:17-18

What is a woman of influence? Today, many admire and follow social media celebrities like Taylor Swift, Beyoncé, Kim Kardashian, or Ariana Grande. But true influence isn't measured by followers or fame—it's measured by character, faith, and the ability to lead with purpose. Lydia was such a woman of influence. She was a leader, a worshiper of God, and someone whose heart was open to the guidance of the Lord. She listened eagerly to Paul's words, allowing her faith to shape not only her own life but also the lives of those around her.

Paul and his companions went to the riverbank in Philippi, where they expected to find a place of prayer, and there they sat among the women gathered. Lydia, a devoted worshiper of God, stood out—her heart open and her spirit seeking truth. When Paul shared the gospel of Jesus, God moved in Lydia's heart, and she became the first recorded convert to Christianity in Europe. Her story reminds us that spiritual openness and a heart willing to seek truth can lead to extraordinary transformation."

"A God-fearing woman named Lydia, a dealer in purple cloth from the city of Thyatira, was listening. The Lord opened her heart to respond to what Paul was saying. After she and her household were baptized, she urged us, "If you consider me a believer in the Lord, come and stay at my house", and she persuaded us."
Acts 16:14-15

Lydia was likely a wealthy, well-known businesswoman during a time when women rarely had such opportunities. She was educated, skilled, and determined to work in a male-dominated society. Therefore, Lydia was clearly an influential and respected person in her family when she and her household were baptized. Additionally, the Lord opened her heart. What does it mean to have an open heart? Lydia was willing to change; she wasn't set in her ways; she didn't go through her life with her head down and her ears closed. She stayed open, and that openness led to her transformation.

When I first heard the gospel, I thought about the sacrifice Jesus made for us. Jesus' crucifixion was proof of God's perfection, His Holiness, His justice, and His love. A debt had to be paid. The disobedience of Adam and Eve in the Garden of Eden resulted in their nature becoming 'fallen,' and sin was inherited by all their descendants. God had a plan for all mankind. He sent His only Son to pay the price for mankind's sins; somebody had to pay for Adam's sin. So, Jesus took it! Took it all! He was already beaten before He was on the cross. Jesus endured the beatings beyond recognition. It was long and painful. A crown of thorns was placed upon His head— the worst death anyone could ever experience. He experienced it. He was betrayed, hated, lied about, and everyone knew He was being falsely accused. He was innocent, and everyone knew He was innocent. He was good, and everyone knew He was good. And they crucified Him anyway. That is the justice of God.

"But He was pierced for our transgressions, He was crushed for our iniquities; the punishment that brought us peace with Him, and by His wounds we are healed. We all, like sheep, have gone astray, each of us has turned to our own way; and the Lord has laid on Him the iniquity of us all."
Isaiah 53:5-6

We deserve that crucifixion. Jesus took that crucifixion. Jesus deserves the love of the Father, and we get the love of the Father. Jesus deserves to be seated at the right hand of the Father. Jesus came to reveal the Father to us.

Jesus tells John the Baptist to baptize Him, saying, "Let it be so now; it is proper for us to do this to fulfill all righteous," (Matthew 3:15). Jesus explains the justification that the baptism is necessary to fulfill all righteous. This is fulfilling God's requirements and completing the mission God sent Him for. Jesus has established a pattern for believers to follow.

It is important to understand Jesus' crucifixion, death, burial, and resurrection. Jesus paid the price for our sins. We do not become righteous because of our goodness or merit; it is through Christ that we are justified in God's eyes because we are identified with Jesus, His Son.

> *"For the wages of sin is death, but the free gift of God is eternal life through Christ Jesus our Lord."*
> *Romans 6:23*

Lydia openly declared her faith to the world. She gathered her entire household, shared what had happened, and as a result, her whole family accepted Christ as their Savior and were baptized. Lydia invited Paul and Silas to stay in her home, visited them, and took care of their needs. Her influence was evident through her generosity, leadership, and obedience to God's calling.

Questions:

1. What about Lydia's conversion teaches us?

2. Why was this courageous? And how can we apply this lesson to our lives?

REFERENCES

- Bergen, Robert D. "Feeling Forgotten? Hannah in the Bible shows us how to pray and trust God." The New Commentary: 1,2 Samuel, Vol 7 (Nashville: Broadman and Holman Publishers, 1996) 67-69 https://estherpress.com/what-hannah-in-the-bible-teaches-us-today/

- Cardillo, Janet. "Lydia of Thyatira: Courageous Hospitality." She is called Women of the Bible Study Vol. 3. https://www.faithward.org/women-of-the-bible-study-series/lydof-thyatira-courageous-hospitality/

- Celoria, Heather. "Who was Abigail?" CBE International, winter 2012. https://www.cbeinternational.org/resource/who-was-abigail/

- Lucado, Max. "Rahab: When a Checkered Past Meets God's Grace." Ten Women of The Bible: One by One They Changed the World. Grand Rapids, Michigan, 2024, pp.25-45

- Riepma, Alisha Rev. "Anna the Prophet: She Never Stopped Praying." She Is Called: Women of the Bible Study Series Vol 2

- Steiner, Ann. "The story of Ruth as you may never have thought of it before." Active Christianity. https://activechristianity.org/ruth-and-naomi-a-book-of-ruth-commentary/

- Thampy, Donald. "The Little Servant Girl." Voice of Grace, July 17, 2025 https://graceredeemer.com/the-little-servant-girl/

- Witherington, Ben III. "Mary, Simeon, or Anna: Who first recognized Jesus Messiah?" https://www.biblicalarchaeology.org/daily/biblical-topics/new-testament/mary-simeon-or-anna-who-first-recognized-jesus-as-messiah/

- Youngblood, Ronald F. (GEN.ED), Bruce, F.F.; Harrison, R.K. (CONS. ED.) (2014). Nelson's New Illustrated Bible Dictionary (Completely Revised).

*"For we are God's masterpiece,
created in Christ Jesus to do good works,
which God prepared in advance for us to do."*

Ephesians 2:10